Negative  Calorie Diet Recipes

Healthy And Nutritious Negative Calorie Meals For Easy Weight Loss

Table of Contents

Introduction

This book contains a wide variety of breakfast, main dish, side dish, and dessert recipes for the Negative Calorie Diet.

The Negative Calorie Diet works because it sticks to the basic rule of weight loss, which is actually quite simple: *eat less and exercise more*. You will definitely lose the extra weight if your body can burn more calories than it consumes, hence the Negative Calorie Diet.

To make this diet work for you, it is highly recommended that you choose a moderate to high intensity workout regimen that you absolutely should stick to on a regular basis.

Along with that, you should create a meal plan composed of dishes that are low in calories but dense in fiber. This is where this book can help you out. Choose from the different recipes here to easily make your Negative Calorie Diet meal plan. For even faster weight loss, substitute the oils that are called for in the recipes with plain old water. However, you don't have to sacrifice healthy oils so long as you work out, because the body still needs good fat to absorb certain nutrients.

Get started on the Negative Calorie Diet immediately. The sooner you begin, the sooner you'll lose weight and feel healthier than you've ever been before.

Let's begin the journey.

Chapter 1: Breakfast Recipes

Could there really be foods that contain zero calories? The truthful answer is: No, unless you're planning on consuming only water and unsweetened tea for the rest of your life. However, the Negative Calorie Diet got its name because it is actually a diet that combines daily exercise with eating foods that are low in calories but high in fiber and nutrients.

Most of all, it is crucial to start your day with a negative calorie breakfast meal. If you don't, you will be giving in to fattening food cravings later on during the morning. The best thing to do each morning is to do a quick, energizing workout, after which you should then enjoy any of these tasty yet super low calorie meals with a hot cup of black coffee or green tea. Doing so will quickly bring you closer to your goal weight.

Oatmeal Muffins

Number of Servings: 18 muffins

You will need:

1. 4 ¼ cups traditional oats

2. 1 ½ tsp ground cinnamon

3. 1 ½ tsp baking powder

4. ¾ tsp ground nutmeg

5. 3 large egg whites, beaten

6. 1/3 cup applesauce, unsweetened

7. 3 Tbsp honey

8. 3 tsp vanilla extract

9. 1/3 tsp fine sea salt

10. 1 ¾ cups non-fat or vegan milk

11. Optional: 1/3 cup brown sugar

How to Make:

1. Set the oven to 350 degrees F. line 18 muffin cups with paper liners and set aside.

2. Combine the egg whites, applesauce, vanilla extract, and honey in a large bowl. Fold in the oats, cinnamon, nutmeg, and baking powder.

3. Gradually stir in the milk until the mixture is thoroughly combined.

4. Divide the mixture among the muffin cups and top each with a bit of brown sugar, if desired.

5. Bake for 25 minutes, or until the muffins are cooked through. Stick a toothpick in the center of one muffin; if it comes out clean, they are done.

6. Set on a cooling rack for about 12 minutes, then take them out of the cups and serve.

Spring Scramble

Number of Servings: 2

You will need:

- ½ tsp olive oil

- 6 egg whites, beaten

- 8 asparagus stalks, trimmed and chopped on the diagonal

- 16 fresh snow pea pods, trimmed and chopped

- 2 green onions, chopped

How to Make:

1. Boil some water in a small steamer pot. Place the chopped asparagus and snow pea pods in the steamer basket, then steam for about 3 minutes or until tender.

2. Drain the asparagus and snow pea pods thoroughly, then set aside.

3. Whisk the egg whites until foamy, then set aside.

4. Place a nonstick frying pan over medium flame and heat through. Once hot, add the olive oil and swirl to coat.

5. Pour the asparagus and snow pea pods into the pan and sauté until crisp tender. Sprinkle in the green onion and mix well.

6. Pour in the egg whites and scramble until set to a desired consistency. Transfer to a plate and serve right away.

Veggie Basil Egg Whites

Number of Servings: 3

You will need:

- 6 egg whites

- 1 ½ cups chopped fresh spinach

- 3 Tbsp chopped fresh basil leaves

- 2 celery ribs, diced

- 6 fresh tomatoes, chopped

- 3 tsp freshly squeezed lemon juice

- Fine sea salt

- Freshly ground black pepper

How to Make:

1. Combine the basil, celery, tomatoes, and lemon juice in a bowl. Season with salt and pepper.

2. Beat the egg whites in another bowl, then set aside.

3. Place a nonstick frying pan over medium heat and heat through. Once hot, stir in the spinach until wilted. Set aside.

4. Rinse and wipe the frying pan, then reheat on medium flame. Pour in the egg whites and reduce to low flame.

5. Add the tomato mixture and spinach on top, then scramble. Transfer to a plate and serve at once.

Bean Sprout Scramble

Number of Servings: 2

You will need:

- 3 Tbsp butter
- 2 Tbsp minced onion
- 1 cup bean sprouts
- 6 egg whites
- Fine sea salt
- Freshly ground black pepper

How to Make:

1. Place a nonstick frying pan over medium flame and heat through. Once hot, add the butter and onion. Sauté until onion becomes tender and translucent.

2. Stir in the bean sprouts and sauté until crisp tender. Pour in the egg whites and scramble to a desired consistency.

3. Season to taste with salt and pepper, then serve right away.

Mushroom and Sweet Potato Hash Browns

Number of Servings: 2

You will need:

- 2 tsp canola oil

- 2 cups chopped mushroom

- 2 cups chopped sweet potato

- 2 garlic cloves, minced

- 2 green onions, chopped

- 1 tsp fine sea salt

- ½ tsp freshly ground black pepper

How to Make:

1. Place a frying pan over medium high flame and heat through. Once hot, add the canola oil and swirl to coat.

2. Stir in the garlic and sauté until fragrant. Add the sweet potato and sauté for about 5 minutes, or until tender.

3. Stir in the mushrooms, then season with salt and pepper. Sauté for 8 minutes, or until everything is browned and tender.

4. Transfer the hash browns into a bowl, then top with green onion and serve right away.

Veggie Breakfast Tortilla

Number of Servings: 3

You will need:

- 1 Tbsp olive oil

- 2 cups finely chopped cauliflower

- 1 small turnip, peeled and thinly sliced

- 1 small onion, thinly sliced

- 6 egg whites

- Fine sea salt

- Freshly ground black pepper

How to Make:

1. Boil water in a small steamer pot. Place the cauliflower and turnip into the steamer basket. Steam for about 6 minutes or until tender.

2. Drain the cauliflower and turnip thoroughly, then set aside.

3. Place a nonstick frying pan over medium flame and heat through. Once hot, add the olive oil and swirl to coat.

4. Add the steamed cauliflower and turnip, then sauté until crisp tender. Reduce to low flame and spread the veggies into an even layer on the pan.

5. Whisk the egg whites and pour on top of the vegetables. Season lightly with salt and pepper. Cover and cook until the egg whites are set.

6. Invert the pan over a plate, slice into wedges, then serve right away.

Pink and Green Smoothie

Number of Servings: 2

You will need:

- 1 cup frozen strawberries

- 2 cups baby spinach

- ½ cup chopped broccoli florets, steamed and cooled

- 2 green onions

- 1 cup freshly squeezed orange juice

- 2 Tbsp ground flaxseed

- 4 tsp honey

- 6 ice cubes

How to Make:

1. In a high power blender, mix together the orange juice, green onion, and spinach. Blend until smooth.

2. Add the rest of the ingredients, then blend again until smooth.

3. Pour the smoothie into two tall glasses, then serve right away.

Banana and Blueberry Breakfast Smoothie

Number of Servings: 2

You will need:

*   1 frozen banana, peeled and chopped

*   2 cups frozen blueberries

*   1 cup freshly squeezed orange juice

*   4 Tbsp non-fat Greek yogurt, unsweetened

*   4 tsp honey

*   6 ice cubes

How to Make:

1. In a high power blender, mix together the banana, blueberries, and orange juice. Blend until smooth.

2. Add the yogurt, honey, and ice cubes, then blend again until smooth.

3. Pour the smoothie into two tall glasses, then serve right away.

Bell Pepper, Zucchini and Artichoke Heart Frittata

Number of Servings: 3

You will need:

- 1 ½ Tbsp olive oil

- 1 ½ Tbsp chopped onion

- 1 small garlic, crushed

- 1 small zucchini, diced

- 1 small red bell pepper, diced

- 1 cup canned artichoke hearts, drained thoroughly and chopped

- 2 Tbsp chopped fresh flat leaf parsley

- 6 egg whites

- ½ Tbsp chopped fresh oregano

- Optional: 2 ½ Tbsp grated Parmesan cheese

How to Make:

1. Place an oven-proof skillet over medium high flame and heat through. Once hot, pour in the olive oil and swirl to coat.

2. Sauté the onion, garlic, bell pepper, and zucchini until tender.

3. Add the artichoke hearts and parsley, then sauté until mixed well.

4. Meanwhile, whisk the egg whites well with the oregano and Parmesan, if using.

5. Spread the artichoke mixture in the skillet, then pour the egg whites on top. Reduce to low flame and cover. Cook until egg whites are set.

6. Prepare the broiler.

7. Once the egg whites are set, transfer the pan into the oven and broil for 2 minutes, or until golden brown.

8. Invert on a plate, slice into wedges, and serve right away.

Fruit and Seed Breakfast Salad

Number of Servings: 3

You will need:

- 2 small apples, cored and chopped
- 2 small pears, cored and chopped
- 2 bananas, peeled and sliced
- 3 cups sliced in-season fruit
- ¾ cup sliced strawberries
- ¾ cup peeled and sliced grapefruit, orange, or other citrus fruit
- ¾ cup berries (such as blueberries, blackberries, raspberries)

- ¾ cup cashews

- ½ cup hemp seeds

- 1 ½ Tbsp freshly squeezed lemon juice

How to Make:

1. Place all of the sliced fruit into a bowl of fruit, then add the hemp seeds and cashews. Toss gently to combine.

2. Pour the lemon juice over the salad and toss again to combine. Serve right away or serve chilled.

Pineapple Floats

Number of Servings: 2

You will need:

- 1 pineapple

- 1 cup sliced banana

- ½ cup halved seedless green grapes

- 1 tsp poppy seeds

How to Make:

1. Halve the pineapple lengthwise starting from the crown and working your way down through the stem. Do not remove the crown.

2. Cut out and discard the pineapple core, then loosen the pineapple flesh from the "shells" by slicing through to the rind and slicing into small pieces. Do not cut the "shells."

3. Transfer the pineapple slices into a bowl and add the sliced bananas and grapes.

4. Spoon the fruit mixture into the two pineapple shells and top with poppy seeds. Serve right away.

Cinnamon Honey Porridge

Number of Servings: 2

You will need:

- ½ cup rolled oats
- 1/3 cup applesauce, unsweetened
- 1 tsp ground cinnamon
- ½ Tbsp honey
- 1 cup water
- ½ tsp almond extract
- Fine sea salt

How to Make:

1. Pour the rolled oats into a food processor and grind until fine. Transfer to a saucepan.

2. Add the water and mix well, then place over medium flame and bring to a boil. Once boiling, reduce to a simmer. Let simmer for about 2 minutes.

3. Stir in the honey, applesauce, cinnamon, and almond extract. Add a dash of salt and simmer.

4. Ladle into bowls, then serve right away.

Cherry Cinnamon Brown Rice Porridge

Number of Servings: 2

You will need:

*   ½ Tbsp olive oil

*   ½ cup uncooked brown rice

*   ½ cup dark cherries

*   2 ½ tsp honey

*   ½ tsp freshly grated orange zest

*   2 ½ Tbsp almond milk

*   ¼ tsp vanilla extract

*   ¼ tsp fine sea salt

*   1 ¼ tsp ground cinnamon

How to Make:

1. Cook the brown rice based on package instructions.

2. Once the rice is cooked, fold in the cinnamon, olive oil, orange zest, and salt. Mix well and divide between two bowls. Set aside.

3. Pour the almond milk into a small saucepan and let simmer over low flame. Once simmered, turn off the heat and stir in the vanilla extract and honey.

4. Pour the hot honey and milk mixture over the rice porridge, then serve right away.

Apple and Pumpkin Porridge

Number of Servings: 2

You will need:

- ¼ cup pureed pumpkin

- 1 small apple, cored and sliced thinly

- 1/3 cup pure apple juice, unsweetened

- ¼ cup non-fat yogurt

- ¾ cup rolled oats

- ½ tsp ground cinnamon

- 1/8 tsp ground nutmeg

- ¾ cup water

How to Make:

1. Mix together the oats, nutmeg, and cinnamon in a bowl. Set aside.

2. Pour the water, apple juice, and pureed pumpkin in a saucepan. Place over medium high flame and bring to a boil.

3. Once boiling, reduce to low flame and stir in the oats mixture. Mix well until heated through.

4. Pour the oatmeal into four bowls, then add the sliced apple on top. Spoon the yogurt over the apple layer, then serve right away.

Tropical Island Oatmeal

Number of Servings: 2

You will need:

- 1 ¼ cups traditional rolled oats

- 1 cup coconut milk, unsweetened

- ½ cup water

- ½ cup sliced fresh papaya or mango

- 1 Tbsp toasted shredded coconut, unsweetened

- Fine sea salt

How to Make:

1. Pour the water, coconut milk, and a dash of salt into a small saucepan. Place over medium flame and let simmer.

2. Once simmering, stir in the oats and mix well until heated through. Turn off the heat and cover the saucepan. Set aside for about 3 minutes.

3. Divide the oatmeal into two servings, then place the sliced fruit on top. Sprinkle on the shredded coconut, then serve right away.

Walnut Banana Muffins

Number of Servings: 18 muffins

You will need:

- 3 cups whole wheat flour

- 3 large eggs, beaten

- ¾ cup chopped walnuts

- 2 cups mashed banana

- 3 tsp baking powder

- 1/3 tsp fine sea salt

- ¾ cup non-fat or vegan milk

- 3 Tbsp canola oil

How to Make:

1. Set the oven to 400 degrees F. line 18 muffin cups with paper liners and set aside.

2. Combine the baking powder, salt, and flour in a large bowl.

3. In another bowl, combine the milk, eggs, banana, and oil.

4. Gradually stir the flour mixture into the milk mixture until thoroughly combined. Add the walnuts and fold until evenly distributed.

5. Divide the mixture among the muffin cups.

6. Bake for 20 minutes, or until the muffins are cooked through. Stick a toothpick in the center of one muffin; if it comes out clean, they are done.

7. Set on a cooling rack for about 5 minutes, then take them out of the cups and serve.

Breakfast Parfait

Number of Servings: 2

You will need:

- 1 Tbsp freshly squeezed orange juice
- ½ tsp freshly grated orange zest
- 2 Tbsp raisins
- 1 cup fresh berries (such as blueberries, raspberries, or sliced strawberries)

- ½ tsp vanilla extract

- 2 oz low fat cream cheese, softened

- ¼ cup low fat granola

- 1 Tbsp honey

How to Make:

1. Pour the raisins into a heatproof bowl and set aside.

2. Pour the orange juice into a small pan and place over medium flame. Let simmer.

3. Once simmering, pour the orange juice into the bowl of raisins.

4. Add the vanilla extract, stir and let plump up for about 2 minutes. Set aside.

5. Meanwhile, beat the cream cheese using an electric mixer until smooth. Add the orange juice and raisin mixture, then the orange zest.

6. Prepare two parfait glasses. Spoon half the orange juice and cream cheese mixture into the two glasses, then add half of the fresh berries, then the granola.

7. Repeat the same sequence with the second layer, then add a drizzle of honey on top. Cover and chill, then serve the following morning. Otherwise, serve right away.

Kale Breakfast Wraps

Number of Servings: 2

You will need:

- 1 Tbsp extra virgin olive oil
- ½ cup lacinato kale leaves, chopped
- 4 egg whites
- 1 small yellow onion, minced
- 1 cup thinly sliced cremini mushrooms
- ½ tsp garlic powder
- Fine sea salt
- Freshly ground black pepper
- 1 small ripe avocado, pitted, peeled and sliced thinly
- ¼ tsp freshly squeezed lemon juice
- 2 large whole wheat or gluten free tortillas

How to Make:

1. As soon as the avocado is sliced, add the lemon juice and mix to coat. Set aside.

2. Place a nonstick frying pan over medium flame and heat through. Once hot, reduce to medium low flame and add the olive oil. Swirl to coat.

3. Sauté the onion until translucent, then stir in the mushrooms and sauté until tender.

4. Stir in the kale and sauté until wilted. Transfer everything into a bowl and set aside.

5. Beat the egg whites with the garlic powder in a small bowl. Pour into the same pan and place over low flame. Cook until eggs are set.

6. Add the kale and mushroom mixture on top of the egg whites and sauté until thoroughly combined.

7. Warm the tortillas on a dry nonstick frying pan, then place on a platter. Divide the kale and egg mixture between the tortillas, then add the avocado. Fold into burritos, then serve right away.

Baked Omelet Bites

Number of Servings: 18 pieces

You will need:

- 9 large eggs, beaten

- 1/3 cup diced onion

- 1/3 cup non-fat or vegan milk

- ¾ cup finely chopped mushrooms

- 4 ½ Tbsp freshly grated Parmesan cheese

- ¾ tsp fine sea salt

- 1/3 tsp freshly ground black pepper
- Nonstick cooking spray

How to Make:

1. Set the oven to 375 degrees F. Lightly coat 18 muffin cups with nonstick cooking spray.

2. In a bowl, mix together all of the ingredients until thoroughly combined. Pour into the prepared muffin cups.

3. Bake for about 15 minutes, or until puffed and cooked through.

4. Stick a toothpick in the center of one cup; if it comes out clean, they are done.

5. Set on a cooling rack for about 3 minutes, then take them out of the cups and serve.

Blueberry Lemon Muffins

Number of Servings: 18 muffins

You will need:

- 3 cups whole wheat flour
- 3 Tbsp freshly squeezed lemon juice
- 1 ½ cups non-fat or vegan milk
- 2 cups fresh blueberries

- 3 tsp baking powder

- 1/3 tsp fine sea salt

- 3 large eggs, beaten

- 1 ½ tsp freshly grated lemon zest

How to Make:

1. Set the oven to 400 degrees F. line 18 muffin cups with paper liners and set aside.

2. Combine the baking powder, salt, and flour in a large bowl.

3. In another bowl, combine the milk, eggs, lemon juice, and oil.

4. Gradually stir the flour mixture into the milk mixture until thoroughly combined. Add the lemon zest and blueberries, then fold until evenly distributed.

5. Divide the mixture among the muffin cups.

6. Bake for 20 minutes, or until the muffins are cooked through. Stick a toothpick in the center of one muffin; if it comes out clean, they are done.

7. Set on a cooling rack for about 5 minutes, then take them out of the cups and serve.

Mushroom and Bell Pepper Omelet

Number of Servings: 2

You will need:

- 1 ½ tsp canola oil
- 6 large egg whites
- 2 Tbsp water
- 4 Tbsp diced onion
- 4 Tbsp diced mushroom
- 1 red bell pepper, seeded and diced
- 2 green onions, chopped
- ¾ tsp fine sea salt
- 1/3 tsp freshly ground black pepper

How to Make:

1. Beat the egg whites with the salt and pepper in a bowl and add the water. Mix well.

2. Place a large nonstick frying pan over medium flame and heat through. Once hot, add the oil and swirl to coat.

3. Add the egg mixture and swirl the pan. Cook until egg starts to set, then loosen the edges and lift to let the liquid whites flow beneath the set part. Cook until the omelet is almost completely set.

4. Add the diced vegetables on half the omelet and fold the other half over it.

5. Flip and cook for 1 minute, then place on a serving platter. Serve right away.

Chia Chocolate Pudding

Number of Servings: 2

You will need:

- ½ Tbsp high quality maple syrup

- 1 ½ Tbsp almond butter, unsweetened

- ½ cup light coconut milk

- ½ cup almond milk, unsweetened

- 1 Tbsp chopped dark chocolate

- ¼ cup chia seeds

How to Make:

1. Combine the almond butter and maple syrup in a small bowl and mix well.

2. Gradually pour in the almond milk until well incorporated, then do the same for the coconut milk.

3. Stir in the chia seeds and chopped dark chocolate, then pour into two clean mason jars.

4. Seal and refrigerate overnight or for a minimum of 3 hours. Serve chilled the following morning.

Pineapple Berry Green Smoothie

Number of Servings: 1

You will need:

- 1 cup fresh baby spinach

- 1 cup frozen berries (such as raspberries and blueberries)

- ½ frozen banana, peeled

- ¼ cup non-fat yogurt

- 1/6 cup chopped fresh pineapple

- 2 Tbsp freshly squeezed orange juice, chilled or frozen

How to Make:

1. In a high power blender, mix together the banana, berries, and pineapple. Blend until smooth.

2. Add the yogurt and orange juice then blend again until smooth.

3. Pour the smoothie into one tall glass, then serve right away.

Matcha Tea Crepes

Number of Servings: 4 crepes

You will need:

- ½ cup almond milk, unsweetened
- 1 small egg
- 1 Tbsp honey
- ½ tsp vanilla extract
- ½ cup whole wheat or gluten free flour
- ½ Tbsp premium quality matcha powder
- Coconut oil
- Fine sea salt

For the Fillings:

- 1 small banana, peeled and sliced
- ¼ cup fresh berries
- Nonfat Greek yogurt

How to Make:

1. Combine the honey, almond milk, vanilla extract and egg in a bowl.

2. In another bowl, combine the flour and matcha powder with a dash of salt. Gradually fold the milk mixture into the flour mixture until just combined.

3. To cook, place a nonstick pancake griddle over medium flame and heat through. Add just enough coconut oil to coat the griddle.

4. Ladle the batter into the griddle and spread to a thin layer. Cook until golden brown and dry, about 30 seconds per side.

5. Cook the remaining crepe batter, then stack on a plate. Serve with Greek yogurt and fruit.

Apple Cinnamon Granola

Number of Servings: 4 ½ cups

You will need:

- 1 Tbsp hemp protein powder
- ½ Tbsp vanilla powder
- 1 apple, cored
- 1 cup buckwheat
- ¾ cup sunflower seeds
- 1/3 cup unsweetened coconut flakes
- 1/3 cup Brazil nuts
- 1/3 cup almonds

- ¼ cup cashews

- ¼ cup pumpkin seeds

- 8 dates, pitted

- ½ Tbsp ground cinnamon

- ¼ tsp fine sea salt

How to Make:

1. Pour the buckwheat, almonds, pumpkin seeds, and sunflower seeds in a bowl and add enough water to keep them submerged by about an inch.

2. Pour the cashews into a smaller bowl and add enough water to keep them submerged by about an inch.

3. Pour the Brazil nuts into another small bowl and add enough water to keep them submerged by about an inch.

4. Cover the bowls and soak overnight.

5. The following morning, rinse all the soaked nuts and seeds well in a fine mesh strainer. Drain thoroughly.

6. Set the oven to 300 degrees F. Line a baking sheet with parchment paper and set aside.

7. Put the Brazil nuts into a food processor and chop until finely ground. Add the remaining nuts and seeds, then chop until coarsely ground.

8. Add the coconut flakes and blend to mix, then pour into a bowl and set aside.

9. Place the dates, cinnamon, protein powder, vanilla, and salt in the food processor. Chop the apple and add to the mixture. Bend until thick and smooth.

10. Pour the cinnamon apple sauce into the bowl of nuts and seeds and mix well until evenly incorporated.

11. Spread the mixture onto the prepared baking sheet and bake for 15 minutes or until the granola is crisp; watch closely to prevent burning.

12. Carefully transfer to a cooling rack and allow to cool before breaking into pieces and storing in an airtight glass container.

Overnight Muesli

Number of Servings: 2

You will need:

- ¾ cup traditional rolled oats

- ½ cup freshly squeezed orange juice

- ½ cup non-fat Greek yogurt

- 2 Tbsp shredded coconut, unsweetened

- 2 Tbsp dried cranberries, unsweetened

- ¼ cup raw pepitas

- ¼ cup chopped almonds

- 1 small red apple

- Nutmeg

How to Make:

1. Pour the oats and juice into an airtight jar, ensuring the oats are completely soaked. Seal tightly and refrigerate overnight.

2. The following morning, transfer the oats into a bowl and fold in the cranberries, shredded coconut, pepitas, and almonds.

3. Core the apple, then slice into small cubes. Fold into the muesli. Add the yogurt and mix well. Add a dash of nutmeg, Serve right away or chill before serving.

Chapter 2: Main Dish Recipes

A main dish does not have to be full of calories for it to be satisfying, because what matters more is that it is full of fiber and nutrients. That way, your stomach will get full easily and stay satiated for several hours until your next meal.

These main dish recipes are easy to make and pair well with any of the side dishes in this cookbook. Prepare them in advance during the weekends, if you wish, so that you can simply reheat them on the stovetop or microwave for an easy lunch or dinner on busy days.

Zesty Chicken and Black Bean Salad

Number of Servings: 2

You will need:

- ½ Tbsp olive oil
- 6 oz boneless, skinless chicken, chopped into strips
- 7.5 oz canned black or pinto beans, rinsed and drained thoroughly
- 1 large orange
- 1 small garlic clove, minced
- 1 small red onion, sliced thinly
- 2 cups mixed salad greens
- 2 Tbsp chopped fresh cilantro
- 1 Tbsp of freshly squeezed orange juice
- 1 Tbsp of freshly squeezed lime juice
- 1 Tbsp extra virgin olive oil
- ¼ tsp ground cumin
- ¼ tsp chili powder
- Fine sea salt
- Cayenne pepper

How to Make:

1. Pour the lime and orange juices into a small jar and add the extra virgin olive oil, cilantro, garlic, and a dash of salt. Seal tightly and shake vigorously. Refrigerate until ready to use.

2. Place a frying pan over medium flame and heat through. Once hot, add the olive oil and swirl to coat.

3. Stir in the cumin, chili powder, a pinch of cayenne and a dash of salt. Stir until fragrant.

4. Add the chicken strips and sauté for about 4 minutes or until cooked through. Transfer to a large bowl.

5. Add the beans and red onion to the chicken. Peel the orange and slice into segments, then add to the salad. Shake the dressing in the jar again, then pour over the salad and toss well to coat.

6. Divide the lettuce between two plates, then add the chicken salad on top. Serve right away.

Shrimp and Veggie Curry

Number of Servings: 2

You will need:

- 6 oz shrimp, peeled and deveined

- 2 tsp olive oil

- 1 cup chopped onion

- 2 tsp minced garlic

- 2 tsp freshly grated ginger

- 2 red bell peppers, seeded and chopped

- 2 carrots, peeled and chopped

- 1 cup chopped mushrooms

- 2 Tbsp curry powder

- 1 ½ cups vegetable broth

- 1 cup coconut milk, unsweetened

How to Make:

1. Wash the shrimp thoroughly, then blot dry with paper towels. Set aside.

2. Place a saucepan over medium high flame and heat through. Once hot, add the olive oil and swirl to coat.

3. Sauté the onion, garlic, and ginger until fragrant, then add the bell pepper, carrot, and mushrooms. Sauté until tender.

4. Add the curry powder, vegetable broth, and coconut milk. Stir until simmering.

5. Add the shrimp, cover, and reduce to low flame. Simmer for 20 minutes, or until the shrimp is cooked through. Serve right away.

Spinach and Strawberry Chicken Salad

Number of Servings: 2

You will need:

- ¾ lb skinless, boneless chicken breast, chopped into thin strips
- 1 ½ cups baby spinach
- 1 ½ cups watercress
- 1 cup halved strawberries
- 2 Tbsp toasted chopped pecans
- 1 small garlic clove, minced
- 1 small red onion, sliced thinly
- 2 Tbsp chopped fresh cilantro
- 1 Tbsp of freshly squeezed orange juice
- 1 Tbsp of freshly squeezed lime juice
- 1 Tbsp extra virgin olive oil
- ¼ tsp ground cumin
- ¼ tsp chili powder
- Fine sea salt
- Cayenne pepper

How to Make:

1. Pour the lime and orange juices into a small jar and add the extra virgin olive oil, cilantro, garlic, and a dash of salt. Seal tightly and shake vigorously. Refrigerate until ready to use.

2. Place a frying pan over medium flame and heat through. Once hot, add the olive oil and swirl to coat.

3. Stir in the cumin, chili powder, a pinch of cayenne and a dash of salt. Stir until fragrant.

4. Add the chicken strips and sauté for about 4 minutes or until cooked through. Transfer to a large bowl.

5. Shake the dressing in the jar again, then pour over the salad and toss well to coat.

6. Divide the spinach, watercress and strawberries between two plates. Shake the dressing in the jar again and pour over the salad and toss well to coat.

7. Add the chicken on top then sprinkle with the pecans. Serve right away.

Zesty Shrimp Salad

Number of Servings: 2

You will need:

- 2.5 oz mixed baby salad greens

- 6 oz shrimp, peeled and deveined

- ¼ small red onion, chopped

- 1 Tbsp freshly squeezed lemon juice

- 1 ½ Tbsp olive oil

- ¼ tsp Cajun seasoning

How to Make:

1. Place a nonstick frying pan over medium high flame and heat through. Once hot, add ½ tablespoon of olive oil and swirl to coat.

2. Add the shrimp and cook for 4 minutes per side or until pink and cooked through. Transfer to a plate lined with paper towels and let drain.

3. Once drained, transfer the shrimp into a bowl and add the red onion and greens. Toss to combine.

4. Pour the lemon juice, remaining olive oil, and Cajun seasoning into a small jar. Seal tightly and shake vigorously.

5. Pour the dressing over the salad and toss to coat. Serve right away.

Bacon Spinach Salad

Number of Servings: 2

You will need:

- 6 cups fresh baby spinach

- 2 thin slices fresh bacon, chopped

- ½ cup thinly sliced red onion

- 1 cup halved cherry tomatoes

For the dressing:

- 2 Tbsp red wine vinegar

- 2 Tbsp minced shallots

- Dry mustard

- Freshly ground black pepper

How to Make:

1. Place a frying pan over medium high flame and heat through. Once hot, add the bacon and cook to a crisp. Transfer to a plate lined with paper towels and set aside.

2. Wipe the frying pan clean with paper towels, then pour in the red wine vinegar and shallot.

3. Add a generous pinch of dry mustard and black pepper. Simmer, stirring frequently, until heated through. Turn off the heat and set aside.

4. Toss the spinach, cherry tomatoes, and red onion in a salad bowl. Spoon the dressing on top, then toss again.

5. Scatter the crisp bacon over the salad, then serve right away.

Roasted Squash and Mushroom Orzo

Number of Servings: 6

You will need:

- 1 ½ Tbsp olive oil

- 1 ½ lb butternut squash, peeled, seeded and chopped

- 4 ½ cups chopped cremini mushrooms

- 1 ½ large onions, quartered

- 3 garlic cloves, minced

- 1 ½ Tbsp chopped fresh oregano or rosemary

- 42 oz vegetable or chicken broth, low sodium

- 2 cups dried whole wheat orzo pasta

- 1/3 cup chopped toasted walnuts

- Freshly ground black pepper

- Nonstick cooking spray

How to Make:

1. Set the oven to 425 degrees F. Lightly coat a baking dish with nonstick cooking spray.

2. Spread the chopped squash on the prepared baking dish, then season with pepper. Cover, then roast for about 10 minutes.

3. Carefully remove from the oven and uncover. Then, scatter the onion, fresh herbs, and mushrooms on top. Add the oil and toss well.

4. Roast for 18 minutes, uncovered, stirring twice throughout the roasting time.

5. In the meantime, pour the broth into a saucepan and place over high flame. Bring to a boil.

6. Once boiling, reduce to simmer and cover.

7. Lightly grease a saucepan with nonstick cooking spray and place over medium flame.

8. Add the garlic and orzo into the pan and sauté until the orzo becomes pale brown.

9. Gradually pour the simmering broth into the saucepan of orzo, stirring all the time. Keep adding while the orzo absorbs the broth.

10. Once all the broth has been absorbed by the orzo, add the roasted vegetables and gently toss to combine. Serve right away.

Skinny Tuna Melt

Number of Servings: 2

You will need:

- 2 slices whole wheat or gluten free bread
- 1 small ripe tomato, sliced thinly
- 1 small red onion, sliced thinly
- 2 Tbsp minced shallot
- 6 oz chunky light tuna packed in brine, drained thoroughly
- 2 tsp minced fresh flat leaf parsley
- 1 Tbsp freshly squeezed lemon juice
- 1 tsp canola oil
- Fine sea salt
- Freshly ground black pepper

How to Make:

1. Turn on the broiler.

2. Toast the slices of bread in a toaster oven.

3. Mix together the lemon juice, canola oil, parsley, shallot, and tuna in a bowl. Season with salt and pepper to taste, then mix well.

4. Spread the tuna mixture over the toasted bread, then add the sliced tomato and onion on top.

5. Broil the open-faced sandwiches for about 3 minutes, then serve right away, or pack for lunch on the go.

Beany Minestrone

Number of Servings: 3

You will need:

- 1 ¼ cups vegetable broth, low sodium
- 1 small onion, chopped
- 1 small garlic clove, minced
- ½ cup chopped fresh tomatoes
- ½ cup thinly sliced green cabbage
- ¼ cup green beans
- ¼ cup chopped celery
- ¼ cup peeled and chopped carrot
- ¼ cup chopped zucchini
- 4 oz canned kidney beans, rinsed and drained
- 4 oz canned chickpeas, rinsed and drained
- 1 ½ cups water
- 1 cup rinsed and shredded spinach
- ¼ cup dry whole wheat or gluten green macaroni pasta

- ¼ tsp dried basil

- Fine sea salt

- Freshly ground black pepper

How to Make:

1. Pour 2 tablespoons of broth into a saucepan and place over medium high flame. Add the onion, garlic, and cabbage and simmer until cabbage is almost wilted.

2. Stir in the rest of the ingredients, except the spinach. Increase to medium high flame and bring to a boil.

3. Once boiling, reduce to a simmer and cover. Simmer for about 10 minutes or until all the vegetables are fork tender.

4. Add the spinach into the soup and stir until wilted. Ladle into soup bowls and serve right away.

Spicy Haddock with Tomato Sauce

Number of Servings: 2

You will need:

- 2 haddock fillets, 4 oz each

- 2 large tomatoes, diced

- 4 Tbsp diced red onion

- 4 Tbsp chopped fresh cilantro

- 4 Tbsp seeded and diced green bell pepper

- 2 Tbsp minced jalapeno pepper, seeded if desired

- 2 Tbsp freshly squeezed lemon juice

- 1 tsp ground cumin

- Cayenne pepper

- Fine sea salt

- Freshly ground black pepper

- Nonstick cooking spray

How to Make:

1. Set the oven to 350 degrees F. Lightly coat a baking sheet with the nonstick cooking spray.

2. Pour the lemon juice over the fillets and season to taste with salt and pepper on both sides.

3. Lay the haddock fillets on the prepared baking sheet and bake for 15 minutes, or until the fillets are cooked through.

4. Meanwhile, place the tomato, red onion, bell pepper, cilantro, and jalapeno in a nonstick frying pan.

5. Place over medium high flame and sauté until wilted and heated through, then season with a pinch of cayenne.

6. Once the fillets are cooked, place them on a serving dish and add the tomato sauce on the side. Serve right away.

Summer Medley Soup

Number of Servings: 2

You will need:

- ¼ Tbsp canola oil

- 1 small onion, chopped

- 1 celery stalk, chopped

- 1 small yellow squash, sliced thinly

- 1 medium zucchini, sliced thinly

- ¼ cup fresh or frozen green beans

- ¼ cup chopped fresh green beans

- 2 cups vegetable broth, los sodium

- 1 plum tomato, peeled and chopped

- 2 Serrano chilies, stemmed and seeded, chopped

- 2 Tbsp chopped fresh cilantro

- Fine sea salt

- Freshly ground black pepper

How to Make:

1. Place a frying pan over medium flame and heat through. Once hot, add the oil and swirl to coat.

2. Sauté the onion, celery, and chili until tender.

3. Stir in the yellow squash, zucchini, beans, and peas for 2 minutes. Pour in the broth, then bring to a boil.

4. Once boiling, reduce to a simmer. Let simmer for about 10 minutes or until veggies are almost tender.

5. Add the tomatoes with their juices and simmer for an additional 8 minutes. Season to taste with salt and pepper.

6. Stir in the cilantro, then ladle into soup bowls and serve right away.

Stir Fried Beef and Bok Choy

Number of Servings: 3

You will need:

- 1 ½ tsp olive oil

- 9 oz sirloin steak, fat trimmed

- 3/3 lb bok choy

- 3 large carrots, peeled and julienned

- 3 Tbsp rice wine vinegar

- 1 ½ Tbsp tamari or light soy sauce

- 3 tsp oyster sauce

- 1 ½ tsp cornstarch

- 1 ½ tsp red pepper flakes

How to Make:

1. Wash the bok choy thoroughly, then drain and chop into bite-sized pieces. Set aside in a colander.

2. Trim excess fat from the sirloin, then slice as thinly as possible with a sharp knife. Set aside.

3. In a bowl, combine the tamari or soy sauce, rice wine, oyster sauce, red pepper flakes, and cornstarch. Mix well.

4. Place a wok over high flame and heat through. Once hot, add the oil and swirl to coat. Reduce to medium high flame.

5. Stir in the beef and sauté until cooked through. Transfer to a plate lined with paper towels and set aside.

6. In the same wok, sauté the carrot and bok choy until bok choy wilts. Add the sauce and sauté until thoroughly combined.

7. Return the beef into the wok and stir fry until heated through. Transfer to a serving dish and serve right away.

Easy Paella Valenciano

Number of Servings: 3

You will need:

- ½ tsp olive oil

- 1 small onion, chopped

- 2 cups vegetable broth, low sodium

- ¾ cup uncooked brown rice

- ¼ lb boneless, skinless chicken breast, fat trimmed

- 12 littleneck clams, scrubbed and rinsed thoroughly

- ½ lb large shrimp, peeled and deveined

- ½ cup fresh or frozen green peas

- 2 Tbsp diced pimientos

- 3 black olives, rinsed and sliced

- 1 fresh parsley sprig, chopped

- Fine sea salt

- Freshly ground black pepper

How to Make:

1. Lightly coat a soup pot with nonstick cooking spray. Place over medium flame and heat through.

2. Stir in the onions until browned and tender. Stir in the broth and increase flame. Bring to a boil, then reduce to a simmer.

3. Add the rice and chicken, then stir well to combine. Add the parsley and season with salt and pepper.

4. Cover and simmer over medium low flame for about 15 minutes.

5. Stir in the clam, shrimp, peas, olives, and pimientos. Stir, then cover and simmer for about 10 minutes, or until rice is completely tender and chicken is cooked through.

6. Remove and throw away unopened clams, then transfer the paella into a serving platter and serve right away.

Chicken Mulligatawny Soup

Number of Servings: 2

You will need:

- ¾ cup cooked shredded lean chicken, boneless and skinless
- 1 ¾ cups vegetable broth, low sodium
- 1 small onion, chopped
- 1 cup chopped tomato
- 1 small carrot, peeled and diced
- 1 small celery rib, diced
- ½ bay leaf
- 1/3 cup cooked brown and/or black rice
- ¾ Tbsp whole wheat or gluten free flour
- ½ Tbsp curry powder
- 2 Tbsp chopped fresh flat leaf parsley
- 2 Tbsp non-fat yogurt
- 1/3 cup non-fat milk
- Cayenne powder
- Ground nutmeg
- Fine sea salt
- Freshly ground black pepper

How to Make:

1. Place a saucepan over medium low flame and add 1 tablespoon of broth. Add the onion and simmer until translucent.

2. Add the curry powder, flour, and a dash of cayenne and nutmeg. Stir well until combined. Add ¼ cup of broth and stir until combined.

3. Increase to medium flame, then stir in the remaining broth, then the carrot, celery, cooked rice, bay leaf, and the tomatoes with their juices. Simmer for about 8 minutes or until the mixture is thickened.

4. Reduce to low flame and cover. Let simmer for about 10 minutes or until the celery and carrot are tender.

5. Stir in the chicken and cook until hot. Season to taste with salt and pepper, then stir in the milk; do not bring to a boil.

6. Ladle the soup into soup bowls and top with yogurt and parsley. Serve right away.

Apple, Jicama, and Carrot Salad with Beef

Number of Servings: 2

You will need:

- 1 Tbsp olive oil

- 1 Tbsp white wine vinegar

- 2 ½ Tbsp pure apple juice, unsweetened

- 3 cups lettuce

- 1 medium apple, cored and sliced thinly

- 1 medium carrot, peeled and julienned

- 1 medium jicama, peeled and julienned

- ½ cup halved fresh pitted sweet cherries

- 4 oz cooked lean beef, sliced into thin strips

- Fine sea salt

- Freshly ground black pepper

How to Make:

1. Pour the oil, vinegar, and apple juice in a small jar and seal tightly. Shake vigorously, then set aside.

2. Divide the lettuce between two plates, then spoon the cooked beef on top.

3. Lay the apples, jicama, carrot, and cherries on top, then shake the dressing again and lightly drizzle over the salad.

4. Season to taste with salt and pepper, then serve right away.

Savory Quinoa Burger

Number of Servings: 4

You will need:

- ½ tsp canola oil

- 1 small red onion, minced

- ½ Tbsp minced garlic

- ¾ cup water

- ¼ cup dry quinoa

- 7.5 oz canned white cannellini beans, rinsed and drained

- ¼ cup chopped fresh cilantro

- 4 whole wheat or gluten free sandwich buns

- ¼ tsp fine sea salt

- 1/8 tsp freshly ground black pepper

How to Make:

1. Pour the quinoa into a fine mesh strainer and rinse several times under cold running water until the water runs clear.

2. Transfer the quinoa into a saucepan and add ½ cup water. Place over high flame and bring to a boil.

3. Once boiling, reduce to low flame, cover and simmer for about 12 minutes or until the quinoa has absorbed all the water. Set aside, covered.

4. Meanwhile, place a frying pan over medium flame and heat through. Once hot, add the canola oil and swirl to coat.

5. Sauté the onion and garlic until onion is translucent, then add the beans, cilantro, salt, pepper, and the remaining ¼ cup water. Simmer for 8 minutes.

6. Turn off the heat and let cool slightly. Then, transfer to a food processor or blender and blend until grainy.

7. Pour the mixture into a bowl and add the cooked quinoa. Mix well, then form into four patties. Refrigerate for about 30 minutes.

8. Prepare the broiler in the oven.

9. Place the quinoa patties on a baking sheet and broil for 5 minutes per side, then slide into warmed sandwich buns and serve right away.

Risotto with Mussels

Number of Servings: 2

You will need:

- 1 tsp olive oil

- 1 small onion, chopped

- 1 small garlic clove, minced

- 12 mussels, scrubbed and debearded thoroughly

- 1 cup water

- ¼ cup dry white wine

- ½ cup vegetable broth, low sodium

- ½ cup uncooked Arborio or brown rice

- 1 Tbsp fresh flat leaf parsley

- Fine sea salt

- Freshly ground black pepper

How to Make:

1. Pour the wine and water into a saucepan and place over medium high flame. Bring to a boil.

2. Once boiling, add the mussels and reduce to a simmer. Cover and cook for about 5 minutes or until the mussels open up.

3. Transfer the mussels into a colander using a slotted spoon. Throw away unopened mussels.

4. Pour the liquid through a fine mesh strainer lined with a cheesecloth and into a bowl. Rinse the saucepan and wipe clean.

5. Pour the strained liquid back into the saucepan, then stir in the broth. Place over low flame and simmer. Season to taste with salt and pepper.

6. Meanwhile, place a nonstick frying pan over medium flame and heat through. Once hot, add the oil and sauté the onion and garlic until tender.

7. Stir in the rice and mix well, then ladle in the hot broth. Stir and gradually ladle in until the rice has completely absorbed all the broth.

8. Fold the mussels into the rice and season to taste with pepper. Fold in the parsley, then serve right away.

Shrimp Salad with Hot Thyme and Garlic Vinaigrette

Number of Servings: 2

You will need:

- 1 Tbsp olive oil

- ¾ lb large shrimp, peeled and deveined with tails intact

- 1 garlic clove, minced

- 1 tsp chopped fresh thyme

- ¾ cup fresh salad greens

- ¾ cup fresh baby spinach

- 2 cups endive leaves, trimmed and chopped

- 1 Tbsp chicken broth, low sodium

- 1 Tbsp white wine vinegar

- 1 Tbsp white wine vinegar

- 2 Tbsp freshly grated Parmesan cheese

- Fine sea salt

- Freshly ground black pepper

How to Make:

1. Wash the shrimp well, then blot dry with paper towels. Season lightly with salt and pepper.

2. Pour the oil into a small saucepan and add the garlic. Place over the lowest possible flame and heat for about 3 minutes.

3. Stir in the vinegar, wine, and thyme and continue to heat over very low flame.

4. In the meantime, place a grill pan over medium high flame and heat through. Once hot, cook the shrimp for 5 minutes per side, or until pink and cooked through.

5. Toss together the salad greens, endive, and spinach. Pour the hot vinaigrette over the greens and toss well.

6. Divide the greens between two plates and lay the shrimp on top. Sprinkle with cheese and serve right away.

Walnut Barley Soup

Number of Servings: 3

You will need:

- 1 Tbsp extra virgin olive oil
- 1/3 cup uncooked hulled barley
- ¾ cup water
- 4 cups vegetable broth, low sodium
- 1 carrot, peeled and diced
- 1 celery stalk, diced
- 1 small yellow onion, minced
- 1 bay leaf
- 2 Tbsp chopped walnuts
- 1 cup shredded lacinato kale leaves
- 1 small ripe avocado, pitted, peeled and sliced
- 1 Tbsp apple cider vinegar
- Nutmeg

How to Make:

1. Pour the water and barley into a soup pot, then place over high flame and bring to a boil.

2. Once boiling, reduce to a simmer. Cook until the barley has completely absorbed the water and is tender. Cover the pot and set aside.

3. Place a saucepan over medium flame and heat through. Once hot, pour in the olive oil and reduce to low flame. Sauté the onion until translucent.

4. Stir in the celery, carrot, and bay leaf. Sauté until the vegetables are crisp tender.

5. Pour in the broth, then let simmer. Add the cooked barley and mix well. Sprinkle in the chopped walnut and a dash of nutmeg. Simmer until heated through.

6. Remove the bay leaf, then fold in the kale. Stir in the apple cider vinegar, then divide among three bowls.

7. Add the sliced avocado on top, then serve right away.

Black Bean Chili

Number of Servings: 3

You will need:

- ½ Tbsp olive oil

- 7.5 oz canned black beans, rinsed and drained

- 7 oz canned stewed tomatoes, low sodium

- ½ tsp minced garlic

- ½ small red onion, diced

- 1 small red bell pepper, diced

- 1 small zucchini, diced

- ½ jalapeno pepper, seeded and minced

- 1 Tbsp chili powder

- ½ Tbsp dried chipotle powder

- ½ tsp dried oregano

- ¼ tsp fine sea salt

How to Make:

1. Place a saucepan over medium flame and heat through. Once hot, add the olive oil and swirl to coat.

2. Add the garlic, chili powder, chipotle powder, and oregano, then sauté until fragrant.

3. Add the onion, jalapeno, and bell pepper, then sauté until onion is translucent and bell pepper is tender.

4. Add the black beans, zucchini, and stewed tomatoes. Let simmer, then cover and reduce to low flame.

5. Simmer for about 20 minutes or until the beans are fork tender. Best served piping hot.

Golden Sweet Potato and Avocado Bowl

Number of Servings: 2

You will need:

- 1 ½ cups uncooked brown rice
- ½ cup roasted cubed sweet potato
- ½ cup shredded curly kale
- 1 small avocado

For the vinaigrette:

- 1 small carrot, peeled and shredded
- 1 Tbsp chopped yellow onion
- 1 tsp rice vinegar
- 1 tsp tamari
- ¼ tsp chopped fresh ginger

How to Make:

1. Combine all the ingredients for the vinaigrette in a blender. Blend well until smooth, then pour into a jar and refrigerate until ready to serve.

2. Cook the brown rice based on manufacturer's instructions.

3. Divide the cooked brown rice between two bowls and add the kale and roasted potato.

4. Halve the avocado, then remove the pit and scoop out the flesh. Slice into small cubes and place on top.

5. Pour the vinaigrette on top, then serve right away.

Broiled Salmon Salad

Number of Servings: 2

You will need:

- 2 fresh salmon fillets, 3 oz each

- ½ cup chopped red onion

- ½ cup chopped tomato

- 4 cups fresh spring greens

- 2 tsp balsamic vinegar

- 2 tsp olive oil

- 2 Tbsp red wine vinegar

- 2 Tbsp freshly squeezed lemon juice

- ½ tsp dry mustard

- 1 tsp freshly ground black pepper

- 1/6 tsp fine sea salt

How to Make:

1. In a small bowl, combine the red wine vinegar, olive oil, balsamic vinegar, black pepper, dry mustard, and salt. Mix well, then set aside.

2. Prepare the broiler and line the rack with aluminum foil.

3. Coat the fillets with lemon juice, then place on the prepared rack. Cook for 5 minutes per side, or until the salmon is cooked to a desired level of doneness.

4. Transfer the salmon on a platter and set aside to cool slightly.

5. Toss together the spring greens, tomato, and onion in a salad bowl. Add the dressing and toss well to coat.

6. Divide the salad between two plates, then place the broiled salmon on top. Serve right away.

Veggie and Salmon Chowder

Number of Servings: 2

You will need:

- 1/3 lb boneless, skinless salmon fillet, chopped

- 1 ¼ cups water

- ½ cup vegetable broth, low sodium

- 1 small carrot, peeled and diced

- ½ small garlic clove, minced

- 1 small onion, chopped

- 1 small celery stock, diced

- 1 medium potato, peeled and cubed

- ¼ cup fresh or frozen green peas

- ½ cup low fat milk

- ½ tsp dried flat leaf parsley

- ¼ tsp dried thyme

- Fine sea salt

- Freshly ground black pepper

How to Make:

1. Pour ¾ cup water into a saucepan and place over medium flame.

2. Add the salmon, cover, and simmer for about 5 minutes or until the salmon is opaque and hot.

3. Transfer the salmon into a bowl using a slotted spoon.

4. Pour the remaining water into the saucepan, then add the remaining ingredients except the milk, salmon, and peas. Increase heat to bring to a boil.

5. Once boiling, reduce to a simmer and cover. Simmer for about 7 minutes or until the vegetables are fork tender.

6. Return the salmon into the saucepan and add the peas. Mix well, then simmer over medium low flame for about 3 minutes.

7. Stir in the milk; do not bring to a boil. Season to taste with salt and pepper, then serve right away.

Thai Inspired Broiled Scallops

Number of Servings: 2

You will need:

- 8 oz bay scallops

- 4 Tbsp of freshly squeezed lime juice

- 2 Tbsp chopped fresh cilantro

- 2 tsp chili powder

- 2 tsp ground chipotle powder

- 1 tsp freshly ground black pepper

- Nonstick cooking spray

How to Make:

1. Wash and drain the scallops, then blot dry with paper towels and set aside.

2. In a bowl, combine the lime juice, cilantro, chili powder, chipotle powder, and black pepper. Mix well.

3. Add the scallops into the marinade, then refrigerate for 20 minutes.

4. Prepare the broiler and lightly coat a roasting pan with the nonstick cooking spray.

5. Place the scallops in the pan about an inch from each other and in a single layer.

6. Broil for about 3 minutes per side or until cooked through. Transfer to a serving plate and serve right away.

Turkey Meatballs in Spicy Sauce

Number of Servings: 3

You will need:

- 1/3 lb lean ground turkey meat

- 1 egg white

- 1 small garlic clove, minced

- ½ small onion, grated

- ½ small carrot, peeled and grated

- ½ Tbsp minced fresh flat leaf parsley

- ¼ cup dry whole wheat or gluten free bread crumbs

- Fine sea salt

- Freshly ground black pepper

- Nonstick cooking spray

For the Sauce:

- 1/3 cup tomato sauce, low sodium

- ½ Tbsp cider vinegar

- ½ tsp dried oregano

- 1/8 tsp cayenne pepper

How to Make:

1. Set the oven to 350 degrees F. Lightly coat a baking sheet using the nonstick cooking spray.

2. Mix together the ground turkey with the bread crumbs, parsley, carrot, onion, and garlic. Season with salt and pepper to taste.

3. Fold in the egg white and mix well until just combined. Divide into 12 small balls, then arrange on the prepared baking sheet.

4. Bake the meatballs for about 30 minutes, or until cooked through and browned all over.

5. Meanwhile, pour the tomato sauce into a small saucepan and place over medium low flame. Stir in the vinegar, cayenne, and oregano. Stir until simmering.

6. Pour the tomato sauce into a platter, then arrange the baked meatballs on top. Serve right away.

Cream of Cauliflower Soup

Number of Servings: 2

You will need:

- 1 tsp unsalted butter

- ¼ cup chopped onion

- 1 small garlic clove, minced

- ¼ cup chopped celery

- 2 cups chopped cauliflower florets

- 2 cups vegetable broth

- ½ tsp dried thyme

- ¼ tsp fine sea salt

- 1/8 tsp freshly ground black pepper

How to Make:

1. Place a saucepan over medium flame and heat through. Once hot, add the butter and garlic and stir until garlic is fragrant.

2. Add the onion and celery, then sauté until celery is tender.

3. Stir in the cauliflower, salt, pepper, and thyme, then sauté for just 1 minute.

4. Pour in the vegetable broth and increase the heat to bring to a boil. Once boiling, reduce to a simmer and cover. Cook for 20 minutes or until the cauliflower is extra tender.

5. Turn off the heat and allow to cool slightly. Puree the solids using an immersion blender, then reheat over low flame and serve. Best served hot.

Savory Clam Soup

Number of Servings: 2

You will need:

- ½ tsp olive oil

- 12 littleneck clams, scrubbed thoroughly and rinsed

- 1 garlic clove, chopped

- ¼ cup chicken broth, low sodium

- 1/3 cup dry white wine

- 1 ½ Tbsp freshly squeezed lemon juice

- 1 Tbsp pimiento, sliced thinly

- ½ tsp crumbled dried thyme

- 1/8 tsp chili pepper flakes

How to Make:

1. Place a soup pot over medium flame and heat through. Once hot, reduce to medium low flame and add the oil. Swirl to coat.

2. Stir in the garlic and chili pepper flakes, then stir until fragrant.

3. Increase to medium high flame and add the broth, wine, lemon juice, and thyme. Stir and bring to a boil.

4. Once boiling, add the clams and reduce to a simmer. Cover and cook for about 15 minutes or until the clams have opened. Stir every now and then.

5. Discard unopened clams, then ladle the rest into two bowls using a slotted spoon.

6. Divide the broth between the bowls, then top with pimiento and serve right away.

Crisp Coconut Chicken

Number of Servings: 2

You will need:

- 1 ½ tsp canola oil

- 6 oz skinless, boneless chicken breast

- 4 Tbsp shredded coconut, unsweetened

- 1 Tbsp coconut flour

- Fine sea salt

- Freshly ground black pepper

How to Make:

1. Set the oven to 400 degrees F.

2. Trim excess fat from the chicken, then rinse and blot dry with paper towels. Season to taste with salt and pepper.

3. Lay the chicken breasts in a baking dish and lightly coat with the canola oil.

4. In a plate, mix together the coconut flour and shredded coconut. Sprinkle the mixture all over the chicken until coated.

5. Bake the chicken for about 25 minutes, or until the chicken is cooked through. Serve right away.

Grilled Veggies and Couscous

Number of Servings: 2

You will need:

- 1 ½ Tbsp olive oil

- 2 Tbsp of freshly squeezed lime juice

- 1 summer squash, cubed

- 1 cup cauliflower florets

- ½ small red onion, thickly sliced

- ½ cup couscous

- ¼ tsp ground cumin

- ¼ tsp freshly ground black pepper

- ¾ cup water

- ½ tsp freshly grated lime zest

How to Make:

1. Prepare the grill.

2. Combine the lime juice, cumin, black pepper, and olive oil. Mix well and set aside.

3. Drizzle some of the lime juice and oil mixture over the chopped squash, cauliflower, and red onion, then toss gently to coat.

4. Grill the vegetables over medium flame until tender, about 10 minutes for the cauliflower and 5 minutes for the squash. Transfer to a plate and keep covered.

5. Pour the water into a small saucepan and place over high flame. Bring to a boil, then add the couscous and lime zest. Stir well, then cover and turn off the heat.

6. Let stand for about 5 minutes or until the couscous has completely absorbed the liquid. Fluff with a fork.

7. To serve, spread the couscous on a serving plate and add the vegetables on top. Drizzle the remaining lime juice and oil mixture over the dish, then serve right away.

Chapter 3: Side Dish Recipes

Side dishes in the negative calorie diet are both filling and highly nutritious because they are all plant-based. The best part of all is that they are also full of flavor. So much so that could even treat them as snacks in between meals.

Nevertheless, be mindful of the recommended serving sizes, especially if you are dedicated to losing weight. Of course, if a second serving can't be helped then putting in a few extra rounds at the gym or miles on the track will be well worth it.

Oven-Roasted Golden Raisins and Swiss Chard

Number of Servings: 3

You will need:

- ½ Tbsp olive oil

- 1 Tbsp balsamic vinegar

- ½ lb Swiss chard

- 3 Tbsp golden raisins

- Fine sea salt

- Freshly ground black pepper

How to Make:

1. Set the oven to 350 degrees F. chop the Swiss chard stems off the leaves and chop into small pieces. Chop the leaves into bite-sized pieces.

2. Place the chopped Swiss chard into a bowl and add the olive oil and raisins. Toss well to combine.

3. Transfer the mixture into a small baking dish and cover with aluminum foil. Seal the edges.

4. Bake for 15 to 20 minutes, or until the Swiss chard is a bit wilted. Carefully uncover and drizzle in the balsamic vinegar. Toss to coat.

5. Season to taste with salt and pepper, then serve right away.

Crisp Swiss Chard with Sunflower Seeds and Cubed Apple

Number of Servings: 2

You will need:

- 1 lb Swiss chard, trimmed

- 1 Honeycrisp or Fuji apple, cored and sliced thinly

- 2 Tbsp sunflower seeds

- ½ small red onion, halved and sliced thinly

- ½ Tbsp freshly squeezed lemon juice

- ½ Tbsp extra virgin olive oil

- ¼ tsp fine sea salt

How to Make:

1. Wash the Swiss chard thoroughly, then dry well. Chop the stems and set aside. Roll the leaves together, then chop into thin ribbons. Set aside.

2. Place a nonstick frying pan over medium flame and heat through. Once hot, add the onion and salt, then sauté until tender, adding a bit of water to prevent burning.

3. Stir in the sliced apple and chard stems until tender, then stir in the leaves and sauté until tender.

4. Add the lemon juice and stir well to combine. Transfer to a plate and top with sunflower seeds. Serve right away.

Tomato and Mozzarella Salad

Number of Servings: 2

You will need:

- 2 ripe tomatoes
- ¾ tsp extra virgin olive oil
- 1 tsp dried oregano
- 1 tsp dried basil
- 1.5 oz fresh mozzarella cheese
- Fine sea salt
- Freshly ground black pepper

How to Make:

1. Chop the tomatoes and mozzarella, then place in a bowl and toss well to combine.

2. Add the dried herbs and olive oil, then a dash of salt and pepper. Toss well to coat.

3. Cover the bowl and refrigerate for at least 1 hour before serving. Best served chilled.

Lentil and Mushroom Soup

Number of Servings: 3

You will need:

- ½ Tbsp olive oil
- 1 small onion, thinly sliced
- 1 small garlic clove, minced
- ½ cup green lentils, rinsed thoroughly and drained
- ½ lb small fresh mushrooms, chopped
- 1 cup thinly sliced carrot
- ½ cup chopped celery
- 7 oz vegetable broth, low sodium
- 2 cups water
- 1 cup shredded red or napa cabbage
- Fine sea salt
- Freshly ground black pepper

How to Make:

1. Place a saucepan over medium flame and heat through. Once hot, add the olive oil and swirl to coat.

2. Sauté the onion until translucent, then add the garlic and sauté until fragrant.

3. Add the lentils and stir to combine, then add the mushrooms, celery, carrot, and a dash of salt and pepper. Mix well.

4. Pour in the broth and water, then bring to a boil. Once boiling, reduce to low flame and let simmer.

5. Cover and cook for about 12 minutes, or until the lentils become tender.

6. Ladle into soup bowls and add the shredded cabbage on top. Serve right away.

Pan Roasted Veggies

Number of Servings: 3

You will need:

- 1 ½ Tbsp peanut oil

- 4 oz baby beets, trimmed and halved

- ¼ cup chopped beet greens

- 4 oz fingerling potatoes, quartered

- 1 small sweet potato, peeled and chopped

- ½ cup trimmed snow pea or snap pea pods

- 2 Tbsp chopped fresh flat leaf parsley or cilantro

- 1 Tbsp freshly squeezed lemon juice

- 1/8 tsp fine sea salt

- Freshly ground black pepper

- 1 lemon, sliced into wedges

How to Make:

1. Place a wok or frying pan over medium high flame and heat through. Once hot, add the peanut oil and swirl to coat.

2. Add the potatoes, sweet potato, and beet. Sauté for about 12 minutes or until fork tender.

3. Season with salt and pepper, then add the pea pods on top and cover. Cook for about 2 minutes, or until the pea pods become crisp tender.

4. Stir in the cilantro, beet greens, and lemon juice, then sauté until combined.

5. Transfer to a serving dish and serve right away with the lemon wedges.

Eggplant Quiniela

Number of Servings: 2

You will need:

- 1 tsp olive oil

- 1 small red onion, sliced thinly

- ½ small garlic clove, minced

- 2 Tbsp dry white wine

- 2 Tbsp dried black currants

- 2 Tbsp red wine vinegar

- 1 small eggplant, diced

- ½ Tbsp honey

- 1 Tbsp chopped fresh flat leaf parsley

- 1 Tbsp chopped fresh or ½ Tbsp dried mint

- Fine sea salt

- Freshly ground black pepper

How to Make:

1. Pour the wine into a small saucepan and add the currants. Place over high flame and bring to a boil.

2. Once boiling, immediately remove from heat and set aside.

3. Place a nonstick frying pan over medium flame and heat through. Once hot, add the oil and swirl to coat.

4. Stir in the onion and sauté until translucent. Stir in the garlic and sauté until fragrant.

5. Stir in the eggplant and sauté until soft, then transfer to a bowl.

6. Pour the currant and wine mixture through a mesh strainer. Set the bowl of wine aside and place the currants into the bowl of eggplants.

7. Pour the wine into the same frying pan and add the honey and vinegar. Place over medium flame and stir until combined and syrupy.

8. Pour the eggplant mixture back into the frying pan and stir until combined. Fold in the parsley and season to taste with salt and pepper.

9. Let simmer, then transfer to a serving dish and serve right away.

Baked Stuffed Tomatoes

Number of Servings: 2

You will need:

- 1 ½ tsp olive oil
- 2 large ripe tomatoes
- 2 garlic cloves, minced
- 1 tsp dried oregano
- 1 tsp dried basil
- 4 Tbsp Italian bread crumbs
- Fine sea salt
- Freshly ground black pepper
- Optional: 2 Tbsp freshly grated Parmesan

How to Make:

1. Set the oven to 350 degrees F.

2. Slice the tops off each tomato, then remove the seeds. Place the tomato on sheet of paper towel, upside down, to drain the insides.

3. Meanwhile, combine the bread crumbs with the dried herbs, garlic, and a pinch of salt and pepper. Add the Parmesan, if using. Mix well.

4. Stuff the tomatoes with the bread crumb mixture, then arrange on a ramekin. Place the tomato tops back on top of each stuffed tomato.

5. Bake for 18 to 20 minutes, or until the tomato is tender. Serve right away.

Caraway Cabbage

Number of Servings: 2

You will need:

- 1 tsp unsalted butter

- ½ lb green cabbage, cored and shredded

- 1 small garlic clove, minced

- 1 Tbsp cider vinegar

- ½ tsp caraway seeds

- ½ tsp honey

- Fine sea salt
- Freshly ground black pepper

How to Make:

1. Place a small saucepan over medium flame and heat through. Once hot, add the butter and swirl to coat.

2. Add the garlic and cabbage and sauté for about 1 minute or until thoroughly combined. Pour in the cider vinegar and mix well.

3. Cover the saucepan and reduce to medium low flame. Allow to cook for about 5 minutes or until the cabbage is wilted.

4. Drizzle in the honey and sprinkle in the caraway seeds. Mix well, then season to taste with salt and pepper. Serve right away.

Cheesy Garlic Broccoli

Number of Servings: 3

You will need:

- ½ Tbsp unsalted butter
- 1 tsp melted butter
- ¾ lb broccoli, chopped into bite-sized pieces
- ¼ cup chopped onion

- 1 garlic clove, minced

- 1 Tbsp whole wheat or gluten free flour

- ¾ cup non-fat milk

- 1.5 oz shredded smoked Gouda cheese

- 1/3 cup soft whole wheat or gluten free bread crumbs

- Fine sea salt

- Freshly ground black pepper

How to Make:

1. Set the oven to 425 degrees F.

2. Boil water in a saucepan or steamer pot. Place the broccoli into the steamer basket and steam over the boiling water, covered, for about 6 minutes.

3. In the meantime, place a saucepan over medium flame and heat through. Once hot, add the unsalted butter, onion and garlic and sauté until the onion is tender.

4. Stir in the flour and season with a bit of salt and pepper. Stir in the milk mix well until sauce becomes thickened.

5. Sprinkle in the cheese as you stir until everything is well incorporated.

6. Place the steamed broccoli into a dry baking dish and pour the sauce on top.

7. Add the bread crumbs and melted butter, then bake for about 8 to 10 minutes, or until the bread crumbs are lightly toasted.

8. Remove from the oven and let stand for about 5 minutes, then serve.

Basil Tomato Soup

Number of Servings: 6

You will need:

- 1 ½ Tbsp olive oil
- 4 large tomatoes, cored
- 2 small onions, chopped
- 2 small garlic cloves, minced
- ½ cup chopped fresh basil leaves
- 3 cups vegetable broth
- 1 tsp fine sea salt
- 2/3 tsp freshly ground black pepper

How to Make:

1. Set the oven to 375 degrees F. Line a baking sheet with baking paper.

2. Halve the tomatoes and place them on the prepared baking sheet. Add the onion, garlic, and basil on top, then add the olive oil.

3. Season with salt and pepper, then roast for about 20 minutes. Shake the pan and roast again for an additional 15 minutes.

4. After roasting, pour everything into a soup pot and add the vegetable broth. Place over high flame and bring to a boil.

5. Once boiling, reduce to a simmer and let simmer for about 12 minutes.

6. If desired, blend the solids until pureed using an immersion blender or food processor. Make sure to let the soup cool slightly before doing so.

7. Ladle into soup bowls and serve right away.

Grecian Vegetable Salad

Number of Servings: 4

You will need:

- 1 Tbsp olive oil
- 1 Tbsp balsamic vinegar
- 1 cup chopped tomato
- ½ cup chopped cucumber
- ¼ cup chopped bell pepper (red, green and/or yellow)
- 1 small red onion, chopped
- ¾ tsp chopped fresh thyme
- ½ tsp chopped fresh oregano
- ½ small head leaf lettuce
- ¼ cup crumbled low fat feta cheese

How to Make:

1. Toss together the tomatoes, cucumber, bell pepper, red onion, and fresh herbs. Set aside.

2. In a bowl, vigorously whisk the balsamic vinegar as you gradually drizzle in the oil. Whisk until thoroughly combined, then pour over the salad.

3. Toss the salad gently to coat in the dressing.

4. Divide the leaf lettuce among four plates, then add the vegetable salad on top. Add the cheese, then serve right away.

Skinny French Onion Soup

Number of Servings: 2

You will need:

- 1 ½ tsp unsalted butter
- 1 large onion, thinly sliced
- 1 small garlic clove, minced
- ½ tsp onion powder
- 2 cups beef broth, low sodium
- ¼ tsp fine sea salt
- 1/8 tsp freshly ground black pepper

How to Make:

1. Place a saucepan over medium high flame and heat through. Once hot, reduce to low flame, add the butter and garlic and stir until fragrant.

2. Add the onion and sauté for about 12 minutes or until caramelized.

3. Add the beef broth and onion powder, then stir well to combine. Increase to high flame and bring to a boil.

4. Once boiling, reduce to low flame and simmer for about 15 minutes. Season to taste with salt and pepper, then serve right away.

Roasted Red Bell Peppers with Capers

Number of Servings: 6

You will need:

- 3 medium red bell peppers

- 1 ½ Tbsp capers, rinsed and drained thoroughly

- 3 tsp minced fresh flat leaf parsley or basil

- 1 ½ Tbsp balsamic vinegar

- 1 ½ tsp olive oil

- Fine sea salt

- Freshly ground black pepper

How to Make:

1. Prepare the grill or broiler.

2. Place the red bell peppers on the grill or broiler pan, then roast for about 15 minutes, turning occasionally, or until the skin is charred and blistered.

3. Place the roasted bell peppers into a brown paper bag and seal. Set aside for about 5 minutes or until cool to the touch.

4. Place a fine mesh strainer over a bowl. Over it, peel the roasted bell peppers to remove the charred skins.

5. Halve the bell peppers, then remove the seeds and stalk. Chop the bell peppers, then arrange on a serving plate.

6. Stir the olive oil into any juice the bowl caught from the bell peppers. Add the balsamic vinegar and capers. Season with salt and pepper, then mix well.

7. Add the chopped herbs and gently mix well. Serve right away.

Grilled Veggie Salad

Number of Servings: 2

You will need:

- 2 tsp olive oil

- 2 ripe tomatoes, halved

- 2 green bell peppers, seeded and quartered

- 1 small red onion, quartered

- 2 cups thickly sliced zucchini

- Fine sea salt

- Freshly ground black pepper

How to Make:

1. Prepare the grill. Line the grate with a sheet of aluminum foil.

2. Put the zucchini, bell pepper, tomato, and red onion in a bowl. Pour the olive oil on top and toss well to coat.

3. Season to taste with salt and pepper, then toss again.

4. Transfer the vegetables onto the lined grate in one layer and grill for 5 minutes per side, turning frequently.

5. Place the vegetables onto a wooden chopping board and chop into bite-sized chunks.

6. Transfer to a bowl, then serve right away.

No-Cook Chili Green Soup

Number of Servings: 2

You will need:

- 6 kale leaves
- 10 lettuce leaves
- 2 celery stalks
- 2 cups warm water
- 1 ½ Tbsp freshly squeezed lemon juice
- ½ mango, peeled and sliced
- 1/6 tsp ground cumin
- 1/3 tsp ground cumin
- 1/3 tsp fine sea salt

How to Make:

1. Place the kale, lettuce, and celery into a high power blender. Pour in the water and blend until smooth.

2. Add the lemon juice, mango, salt, cayenne, and cumin. Blend until well incorporated.

3. Pour the mixture into a serving bowl, then serve right away.

Sun-Dried Tomato and Greens Salad

Number of Servings: 2

You will need:

- 2 sun-dried tomatoes packed in oil

- 2 cups fresh baby spinach

- 4 cups fresh spring greens

- 1 cup halved grape tomatoes

- ½ cup thinly sliced red onion

- ½ cup chopped celery

- 2 garlic cloves

- 2 Tbsp red wine vinegar

- 4 tsp canola oil

- Freshly ground black pepper

How to Make:

1. In a salad bowl, gently toss the spinach and spring greens, then the celery and red onion. Divide between two plates.

2. In a food processor, combine the sun-dried tomatoes, garlic, red wine vinegar, canola oil, and a pinch of black pepper. Blend until smooth.

3. Pour the dressing over the salad and toss to combine. Serve right away.

No-Cook Basil, Avocado, and Carrot Soup

Number of Servings: 2

You will need:

- 2 small carrot, peeled and chopped
- ½ cup fresh basil
- 2 ½ Tbsp walnuts
- ¼ cup sliced avocado
- ½ Tbsp freshly squeezed lemon juice
- ¼ tsp fine sea salt
- 1 ½ cups warm water
- 1 Tbsp hemp seeds

How to Make:

1. Place the carrot, basil, avocado, and lemon juice in a high power blender. Pour in the water, then blend until smooth.

2. Add the walnuts, hemp seeds, and salt. Blend until coarsely ground. Pour into a serving bowl and serve right away.

Hearty Carrot Soup

Number of Servings: 6

You will need:

- 1 ½ Tbsp olive oil

- 3 cups vegetable broth

- 6 cups chopped carrot

- 2 small garlic cloves, minced

- 1 ½ cups chopped onion

- 1 ½ tsp ground turmeric

- 1 ½ tsp dried oregano

- Fine sea salt

- Freshly ground black pepper

How to Make:

1. Place a saucepan over medium flame and heat through. Once hot, add the olive oil and garlic and sauté until fragrant.

2. Add the carrots and sauté until tender, about 10 minutes.

3. Stir in the onion, oregano and turmeric, then sauté for about 4 minutes.

4. Pour in the vegetable broth and let boil. Once boiling, reduce to a simmer and cover. Simmer for 18 minutes or until the carrots are extra tender.

5. Turn off the heat and let cool slightly. Puree the solids using an immersion blender, then reheat over medium low flame.

6. Season to taste with salt and pepper, if needed, then serve right away.

Tender Veggies and Greens

Number of Servings: 3 servings

You will need:

- 1 bunch dark leafy greens (such as spinach, kale, Swiss chard, collard greens)

- 1 small zucchini, diced

- 1 small red bell pepper, cored, seeded and diced

- 1 ½ Tbsp minced onion

- 1 ½ Tbsp freshly squeezed lemon juice

- ¼ tsp fine sea salt

How to Make:

1. Finely chop the leafy greens into thin strips. Place in a large bowl.

2. Add the lemon juice and salt to the greens, then mix well to coat. Lightly squeeze the greens until tender and wilted.

3. Put the diced zucchini and bell pepper into the bowl of greens, then add the onion and toss well to combine. Serve right away.

Carrot and Broccoli Salad

Number of Servings: 3

You will need:

- 2 cups chopped broccoli florets, steamed

- 1 small carrot, peeled and grated

- 1 green onion, chopped

- ¼ cup golden raisins

- ¼ cup slivered almonds

- 2 ½ Tbsp sesame tahini

- 1 ½ Tbsp honey

- ½ tsp freshly squeezed lemon juice

- ½ Tbsp extra virgin olive oil

How to Make:

1. Toss the steamed broccoli, carrot, and green onion in a salad bowl. Add the raisins and almonds and toss well to combine.

2. In a small bowl, whisk together the tahini, honey, lemon juice, and olive oil. Pour the dressing over the salad and toss well to coat.

3. Cover the bowl and refrigerate for at least 1 hour or until chilled. Best served chilled.

Sea Veggie, Celery and Carrot Salad with Pine Nuts

Number of Servings: 2

You will need:

- 1 cup peeled and shredded carrot

- ¼ cup chopped celery

- ½ cup dry arame

- 1 ½ Tbsp of freshly squeezed lime juice

- ½ tsp pine nuts

- 1 Tbsp sesame oil

How to Make:

1. Place the arame in a small bowl, then add enough water to completely soak it. Soak for 1 hour, then drain thoroughly.

2. Rinse the arame, then place in a bowl and add the carrot and celery. Toss well to combine.

3. Add the lime juice, salt, and sesame oil, then toss again to coat. Top with pine nuts, then serve right away.

Cream of Mushroom Soup

Number of Servings: 2

You will need:

- 1 tsp unsalted butter
- ½ lb sliced mushrooms
- 1 small garlic clove, minced
- ¼ cup chopped onion
- 1 ½ cups vegetable broth
- ¼ cup coconut milk
- ¼ tsp salt
- 1/8 tsp freshly ground black pepper

How to Make:

1. Place a saucepan over medium flame and heat through. Once hot, add the butter and garlic and stir until fragrant.

2. Add the onion and stir until translucent. Stir in the mushrooms and season with the salt and pepper. Mix well and sauté until mushrooms are tender.

3. Add the vegetable broth and increase the flame to bring to a boil.

4. Once boiling, reduce to a simmer and cover. Simmer for about 15 minutes.

5. Turn off the heat and let cool slightly. Then, blend the solids using an immersion blender.

6. Add the coconut milk and mix well. Reheat over low flame. Best served warm.

Simple Daikon and Carrot Slaw

Number of Servings: 3

You will need:

- 3 carrots, peeled and shredded

- 2 small daikon radishes, peeled and shredded

- 2 ½ tsp sesame oil

- 4 ½ Tbsp hemp or sesame seeds

- 1 tsp fine sea salt

How to Make:

1. Place the shredded carrot and radish in a bowl, then add the sesame oil and toss well to coat.

2. Sprinkle in the seeds and salt, then toss well to combine.

3. Chill until ready to serve, or serve right away.

Chapter 4: Dessert Recipes

Dessert is usually heavy on the sugar and carbohydrates, which easily makes it a type of food you should avoid if your goal is to lose weight. However, it would do you more harm than good to deprive yourself too much.

You can still enjoy a tasty dessert every now and then in the Negative Calorie Diet so long as you exercise regularly. These delectable dessert recipes call only for the healthiest ingredients so that even your dessert can give you a lot of nutrients.

Tropical Fruit Bowl

Number of Servings: 2

You will need:

- ½ cup chopped fresh pineapple
- 1 orange, peeled and sliced
- 1 small mango, peeled and sliced
- 1 banana, peeled and sliced
- 1 kiwi, peeled and sliced

How to Make:

1. Toss all the fruit together in a bowl and refrigerate until chilled.
2. Divide the chilled fruit between two bowls, then serve right away.

Blueberry Ricotta Cheesecake

Number of Servings: 5

You will need:

- 15 oz low fat ricotta cheese

- 1 egg

- ¾ tsp vanilla extract

- ¼ cup honey

- ¼ cup low fat buttermilk

- ¼ cup evaporated milk, low fat

- ¾ tsp vanilla extract

- ½ Tbsp freshly squeezed orange juice

- ½ Tbsp freshly grated orange zest

- ½ Tbsp chopped toasted almonds

For the Blueberry Sauce:

- ½ pint fresh blueberries, rinsed

- ¾ Tbsp freshly squeezed lemon juice

- ½ tsp honey

How to Make:

1. Set the oven to 375 degrees F. Line a small spring form pan (or ovenproof ramekin) with parchment paper, then set aside.

2. Place the ricotta cheese, vanilla extract, egg, milk, buttermilk, and orange juice in a food processor. Blend until thoroughly combined.

3. Add the orange zest and blend again until combined. Transfer to a bowl, then fold in the chopped almonds.

4. Pour the mixture into the prepared spring form pan, then bake for about 30 minutes or until firm.

5. In the meantime, pour the blueberries into a food processor and add the rest of the sauce ingredients. Blend until the berries are coarsely chopped.

6. Once baked, transfer the cake to a cooling rack and allow to completely cool. Carefully remove the spring form pan sides (or lift the cake from the ramekin), then pour the sauce on top. Serve right away.

Baked Cinnamon Apple

Number of Servings: 3

You will need:

- 3 apples
- 3 Tbsp brown sugar
- ¾ cup apple juice, unsweetened
- ¼ tsp ground cinnamon

How to Make:

1. Set the oven to 350 degrees F.

2. Slice off the apple tops, then core the apples.

3. Arrange the apples on a baking dish and sprinkle the sugar inside the hollow of each.

4. Pour the apple juice around the apples, then sprinkle the cinnamon on top of the apples.

5. Cover the baking dish with aluminum foil, then bake for about 30 minutes or until the apples are crisp tender.

6. Carefully remove from the oven and let stand, covered, on a cooling rack for about 15 minutes.

7. Uncover and serve right away, or chill before serving.

Chocolate Hazelnut Pudding

Number of Servings: 4

You will need:

- ½ cup evaporated milk, low fat
- ¾ cup crumbled chocolate graham crackers
- 1 Tbsp melted unsalted butter
- 1 cup low fat milk
- 3 Tbsp muscovado sugar
- 1 Tbsp cornstarch
- 2 Tbsp cacao powder
- 1 egg
- 1 tsp vanilla extract
- 1 Tbsp chopped hazelnuts
- 1 tsp hazelnut extract
- ¼ oz shaved dark chocolate

How to Make:

1. Set the oven to 375 degrees F.
2. Pour the crumbled crackers in a bowl and add the melted butter. Mix well, then pour into a small pie plate or ramekin and press down to form the crust.

3. Bake the crust for 4 minutes, or until firm. Transfer to a cooling rack. Once cooled, transfer to the refrigerator.

4. Pour the low fat milk, cornstarch, cacao powder, and 2 tablespoons muscovado sugar in a small saucepan. Place over medium flame and stir for 5 minutes or until thickened and hot.

5. Pour 2 tablespoons of the mixture into the egg, then whisk vigorously. Pour the egg mixture into the saucepan of sauce, then stir in the vanilla extract and hazelnut extract. Place over the lowest possible flame and cook, stirring well, until thickened.

6. Pour the mixture into a bowl and place a sheet of plastic wrap on top. Set aside to cool slightly, then refrigerate for at least 3 hours, preferably overnight.

7. Pour the evaporated milk in a bowl, then place the bowl in the freezer for about 2 hours.

8. Remove the evaporated milk from the freezer and blend until stiff.

9. Uncover the chocolate pudding and fold in the evaporated milk. Pour over the crust, then sprinkle the shaved chocolate and chopped hazelnuts on top. Chill, then serve.

Lemon Pudding

Number of Servings: 3

You will need:

- ¾ cup water

- 1/3 cup baking sugar

- 2 ½ Tbsp freshly squeezed lemon juice

- ½ Tbsp freshly squeezed lemon zest

- ¾ Tbsp cornstarch

- 2 small egg yolks

- Fine sea salt

How to Make:

1. Pour the water into a small saucepan and add the sugar. Place over medium high flame.

2. Meanwhile, combine the cornstarch and lemon juice in a bowl and mix well until smooth. Pour the mixture into the saucepan of boiling sugar water.

3. Whisk the egg yolks in a bowl, then pour into the saucepan. Mix well until smooth, then turn off the heat.

4. Add a dash of salt into the saucepan, then stir in the lemon zest. Set aside for 5 minutes or until thickened.

5. Once thickened, pour the pudding into three small ramekins and chill for at least 2 hours. Best served chilled.

Kiwi Raspberry Sorbet

Number of Servings: 12

You will need:

- 4 ½ cups fresh raspberries

- 3 fresh kiwi, peeled

- 4 ½ Tbsp freshly squeezed lemon juice

- 1 ½ Tbsp freshly grated lemon zest

- 3 cups baking sugar

How to Make:

1. Pour all of the ingredients into a food processor and blend until the mixture is smooth and creamy.

2. Pour the mixture into a shallow bowl, then place in the freezer. Freeze for about 1 hour.

3. After an hour, gently stir the mixture, then freeze again for at least an hour or until thick and creamy.

4. Pour the mixture into the food processor and blend again until smooth. Pour into sorbet glasses, then serve right away.

Chiffon Cake

Number of Servings: 6

You will need:

- ¾ cup sifted cake flour
- ¾ cup muscovado sugar
- 1 tsp baking powder
- ½ tsp baking soda
- 1/8 tsp fine sea salt
- 4 egg whites
- ¾ tsp vanilla extract
- 1/8 tsp cream of tartar
- 2 ½ Tbsp low fat buttermilk
- 2 ½ Tbsp safflower oil
- 2 ½ Tbsp warm water
- 1 ½ Tbsp freshly squeezed lemon juice
- ½ Tbsp freshly grated lemon zest

How to Make:

1. Set the oven to 350 degrees F. line a small round cake pan with parchment paper and set aside.

2. Sift the flour into a bowl and add the muscovado sugar, baking soda, baking powder, and salt.

3. In a large bowl, whisk the egg whites vigorously until foamy. Sprinkle in the cream of tartar and whisk until soft peaks form.

4. Pour the oil, buttermilk, water, lemon juice and zest, and vanilla extract into the flour mixture, then gradually fold the flour and buttermilk mixture into the egg whites until combined.

5. Pour the mixture into the prepared cake pan and bake for about 30 minutes or until the cake is cooked through. Insert a toothpick in the center of the cake; if it comes out clean, it is ready.

6. Carefully place the cake on a cooling rack and let cool, then transfer to a plate, slice, and serve.

Simple Banana Foster

Number of Servings: 3

You will need:

- 2 bananas, peeled and sliced lengthwise

- 2 Tbsp brown sugar

- 1 ½ Tbsp water

- ½ Tbsp freshly squeezed lemon juice

- 1 tsp unsalted butter

- ¼ tsp ground cinnamon

- 2 Tbsp crushed graham crackers

How to Make:

1. Set the oven to 450 degrees F.

2. Combine the water, lemon juice, sugar, and cinnamon in a saucepan, then place over medium high flame and let simmer.

3. Once simmering, turn off the heat and add the butter. Mix well.

4. Dip the bananas into the mixture and turn to coat. Transfer everything into a glass baking dish.

5. Top with crushed graham crackers, then bake for about 6 minutes, or until bubbly.

6. Set on a cooling rack and let cool slightly, then serve.

Coco Choco Whole Wheat Cupcakes

Number of Servings: 18 cupcakes

You will need:

- 1 ½ cups whole wheat flour

- 1 ½ cups muscovado sugar

- ¾ cup coconut flakes, unsweetened

- 3 large eggs

- 4 ½ Tbsp low fat milk

- ¾ cup unsalted butter, softened

- 1/3 cup cacao powder

- 1 ½ tsp baking powder

- ¾ tsp vanilla extract

- Fine sea salt

How to Make:

1. Set the oven to 350 degrees F. line 18 cupcake molds with paper liners, or use silicone molds.

2. Mix together the cacao powder with the baking powder and flour. Add a pinch of salt and mix well.

3. In another bowl, blend the sugar and butter with an electric mixer until fluffy. Add the eggs and blend again until smooth.

4. Pour the milk into the egg mixture until smooth, then add the vanilla extract and blend again until combined.

5. Gradually mix the flour mixture into the egg mixture until thoroughly incorporated.

6. Pour the batter into the prepared cupcake molds, then top with coconut flakes.

7. Bake for 20 minutes, or until done. Insert a toothpick into the center of one cupcake; if it comes out clean, they are ready.

8. Set on a cooling rack and let cool before serving.

Spiced Apple Pear

Number of Servings: 4

You will need:

- ¼ cup unbleached all-purpose flour
- 2 Tbsp whole wheat flour
- 2 Tbsp rolled oats
- 1 Tbsp muscovado sugar
- ½ tsp ground ginger
- ¼ tsp ground allspice
- ¼ tsp ground coriander
- ¾ Tbsp unsalted butter

- 1 large pear

- 2 small apples

- 2 Tbsp freshly squeezed lemon juice

- 1 Tbsp thawed frozen apple juice concentrate

How to Make:

1. Set the oven to 375 degrees F. Line a small baking sheet with parchment paper and set aside.

2. In a bowl, mix together the spices, muscovado sugar, oats and flour. Cut in the butter until the mixture becomes crumbly.

3. Core and peel the pear and apples, then slice thinly. Pour the lemon juice over them to prevent them from browning.

4. Place the sliced pear and apples in the prepared pan and add the apple juice over them. Sprinkle the crumbly mixture on top, then bake for about 15 minutes or until the crumbs are golden brown.

5. Transfer to a cooling rack and let stand for about 5 minutes, then serve.

Conclusion

I hope this book was able to help you to prepare delicious and nutritious dishes to supplement your Negative Calorie Diet. Stay motivated to work out regularly and stick to eating healthy whole foods. Always keep in mind the that Negative Calorie Diet works so long as you combine working out well with healthy low calorie meals.

I wish you the best of luck!

Samantha Clare

Made in United States
Orlando, FL
11 November 2021